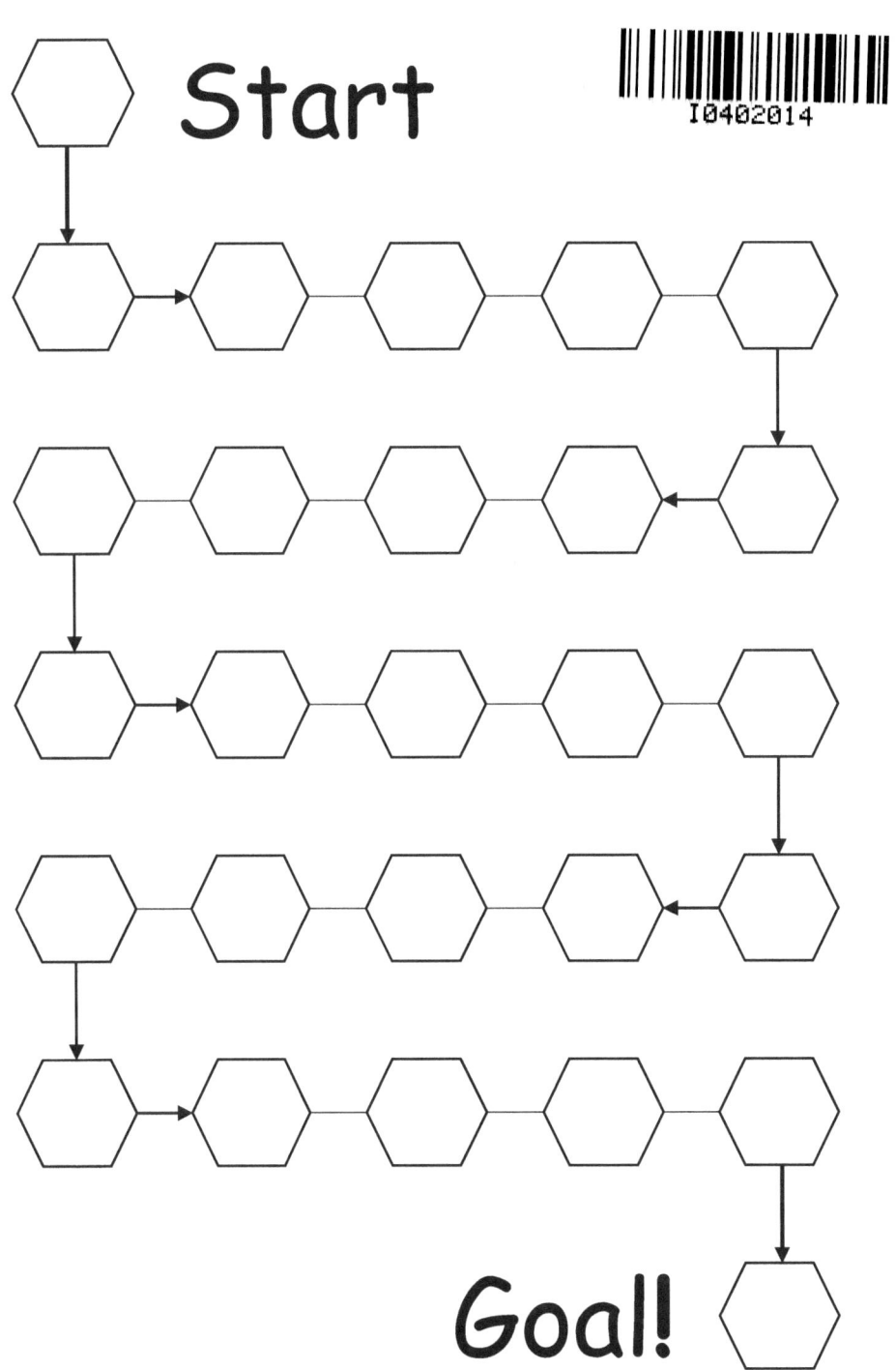

PROGRESS TRACKER

Date:										
chest										
waist										
stomach										
right arm										
left arm										
right leg										
left leg										

Date: ⟶

Weight										

PROGRESS TRACKER

Date:										
chest										
waist										
stomach										
right arm										
left arm										
right leg										
left leg										

Date: ⟶

Weight										

Date: _____

breakfast/lunch/dinner/snacks	carbs	fat	prot.	cal.
Total				

water	🥛 🥛 🥛 🥛 🥛 🥛 🥛 🥛	How do I feel today?		
sleep	zzz zzz zzz zzz zzz zzz zzz zzz zzz	🙂	😐	☹️

activity	sets/reps/distance/time	cal. burned

I am pleased with:	What could be improved:

Date: _____

breakfast/lunch/dinner/snacks	carbs	fat	prot.	cal.
Total				

water 🥛🥛🥛🥛🥛🥛🥛🥛

sleep 💤💤💤💤💤💤💤💤💤💤

How do I feel today? 🙂 😐 ☹️

activity	sets/reps/distance/time	cal. burned

I am pleased with:	What could be improved:

Date: _____

breakfast/lunch/dinner/snacks	carbs	fat	prot.	cal.
	Total			

water ▯▯▯▯▯▯▯▯
sleep 💤💤💤💤💤💤💤💤💤

How do I feel today? 🙂 😐 ☹

activity	sets/reps/distance/time	cal. burned

I am pleased with:

What could be improved:

Date: _____

breakfast/lunch/dinner/snacks	carbs	fat	prot.	cal.
	Total			

water ▯▯▯▯▯▯▯▯▯

sleep zzz zzz zzz zzz zzz zzz zzz zzz zzz

How do I feel today? :) :| :(

activity	sets/reps/distance/time	cal. burned

I am pleased with:	What could be improved:

Date: _____

breakfast/lunch/dinner/snacks	carbs	fat	prot.	cal.
Total				

water	🥛🥛🥛🥛🥛🥛🥛🥛	How do I feel today?
sleep	💤💤💤💤💤💤💤💤💤	☺ 😐 ☹

activity	sets/reps/distance/time	cal. burned

I am pleased with:	What could be improved:

Date: _____

breakfast/lunch/dinner/snacks	carbs	fat	prot.	cal.
	Total			

water | 🥛 🥛 🥛 🥛 🥛 🥛 🥛 🥛

sleep | 💤 💤 💤 💤 💤 💤 💤 💤 💤

How do I feel today? 😊 | 😐 | ☹️

activity	sets/reps/distance/time	cal. burned

I am pleased with:	What could be improved:

Date: _____

breakfast/lunch/dinner/snacks	carbs	fat	prot.	cal.
Total				

water: ☐ ☐ ☐ ☐ ☐ ☐ ☐ ☐
sleep: zzz zzz zzz zzz zzz zzz zzz zzz zzz

How do I feel today? 😊 😐 ☹

activity	sets/reps/distance/time	cal. burned

I am pleased with:	What could be improved:

Date: _____

breakfast/lunch/dinner/snacks	carbs	fat	prot.	cal.
Total				

water	🥛 🥛 🥛 🥛 🥛 🥛 🥛 🥛	How do I feel today?		
sleep	zzz zzz zzz zzz zzz zzz zzz zzz zzz zzz	🙂	😐	☹️

activity	sets/reps/distance/time	cal. burned

I am pleased with:	What could be improved:

Date: _____

breakfast/lunch/dinner/snacks	carbs	fat	prot.	cal.
Total				

water	🥛🥛🥛🥛🥛🥛🥛🥛	How do I feel today?
sleep	💤💤💤💤💤💤💤💤💤	😊 😐 ☹

activity	sets/reps/distance/time	cal. burned

I am pleased with:	What could be improved:

Date: _____

breakfast/lunch/dinner/snacks	carbs	fat	prot.	cal.
Total				

water ☐☐☐☐☐☐☐☐☐☐

sleep 💤💤💤💤💤💤💤💤💤💤

How do I feel today? 🙂 😐 ☹

activity	sets/reps/distance/time	cal. burned

I am pleased with:	What could be improved:

Date: _____

breakfast/lunch/dinner/snacks	carbs	fat	prot.	cal.
	Total			

water	🥛🥛🥛🥛🥛🥛🥛🥛	How do I feel today?		
sleep	💤💤💤💤💤💤💤💤💤	🙂	😐	☹

activity	sets/reps/distance/time	cal. burned

I am pleased with:	What could be improved:

Date: _____

breakfast/lunch/dinner/snacks	carbs	fat	prot.	cal.
Total				

		How do I feel today?		
water	☐ ☐ ☐ ☐ ☐ ☐ ☐ ☐	☺	😐	☹
sleep	zzz zzz zzz zzz zzz zzz zzz zzz zzz zzz			

activity	sets/reps/distance/time	cal. burned

I am pleased with:	What could be improved:

Date: _____

breakfast/lunch/dinner/snacks	carbs	fat	prot.	cal.
	Total			

water	🥛🥛🥛🥛🥛🥛🥛🥛🥛
sleep	💤💤💤💤💤💤💤💤💤

How do I feel today?   😊   😐   ☹️

activity	sets/reps/distance/time	cal. burned

I am pleased with:	What could be improved:

Date: _____

breakfast/lunch/dinner/snacks	carbs	fat	prot.	cal.
	Total			

water ☐ ☐ ☐ ☐ ☐ ☐ ☐ ☐ ☐

sleep 💤 💤 💤 💤 💤 💤 💤 💤 💤

How do I feel today? 🙂 😐 ☹️

activity	sets/reps/distance/time	cal. burned

I am pleased with:	What could be improved:

Date: _____

breakfast/lunch/dinner/snacks	carbs	fat	prot.	cal.
	Total			

water	🥛 🥛 🥛 🥛 🥛 🥛 🥛 🥛	How do I feel today?		
sleep	zzz zzz zzz zzz zzz zzz zzz zzz zzz	🙂	😐	☹️

activity	sets/reps/distance/time	cal. burned

I am pleased with:	What could be improved:

Date: _____

breakfast/lunch/dinner/snacks	carbs	fat	prot.	cal.
Total				

water: ☐ ☐ ☐ ☐ ☐ ☐ ☐ ☐ ☐ ☐
sleep: 💤 💤 💤 💤 💤 💤 💤 💤 💤 💤

How do I feel today? 🙂 😐 🙁

activity	sets/reps/distance/time	cal. burned

I am pleased with:

What could be improved:

Date:_____

breakfast/lunch/dinner/snacks	carbs	fat	prot.	cal.
Total				

water	🥛🥛🥛🥛🥛🥛🥛🥛	How do I feel today?		
sleep	💤💤💤💤💤💤💤💤	🙂	😐	☹️

activity	sets/reps/distance/time	cal. burned

I am pleased with:	What could be improved:

Date: _____

breakfast/lunch/dinner/snacks	carbs	fat	prot.	cal.
	Total			

water ▢ ▢ ▢ ▢ ▢ ▢ ▢ ▢

sleep 💤 💤 💤 💤 💤 💤 💤 💤 💤

How do I feel today? 😊 😐 ☹

activity	sets/reps/distance/time	cal. burned

I am pleased with:	What could be improved:

Date: _____

breakfast/lunch/dinner/snacks	carbs	fat	prot.	cal.
Total				

water	🥛🥛🥛🥛🥛🥛🥛🥛🥛	How do I feel today?		
sleep	💤💤💤💤💤💤💤💤💤	😊	😐	☹️

activity	sets/reps/distance/time	cal. burned

I am pleased with:	What could be improved:

Date:_____

breakfast/lunch/dinner/snacks	carbs	fat	prot.	cal.
Total				

water	☐ ☐ ☐ ☐ ☐ ☐ ☐ ☐ ☐	How do I feel today?		
sleep	zzz zzz zzz zzz zzz zzz zzz zzz zzz	☺	😐	☹

activity	sets/reps/distance/time	cal. burned

I am pleased with:	What could be improved:

Date: _____

breakfast/lunch/dinner/snacks	carbs	fat	prot.	cal.
Total				

water	🥛 🥛 🥛 🥛 🥛 🥛 🥛 🥛	How do I feel today?		
sleep	zzz zzz zzz zzz zzz zzz zzz zzz zzz	😊	😐	☹️

activity	sets/reps/distance/time	cal. burned

I am pleased with:	What could be improved:

Date: _____

breakfast/lunch/dinner/snacks	carbs	fat	prot.	cal.
Total				

water ☐ ☐ ☐ ☐ ☐ ☐ ☐ ☐

sleep 💤 💤 💤 💤 💤 💤 💤 💤 💤

How do I feel today? 🙂 😐 ☹️

activity	sets/reps/distance/time	cal. burned

I am pleased with:

What could be improved:

Date: _____

breakfast/lunch/dinner/snacks	carbs	fat	prot.	cal.
	Total			

water 🥛🥛🥛🥛🥛🥛🥛🥛
sleep 💤💤💤💤💤💤💤💤💤

How do I feel today? 😊 😐 ☹

activity	sets/reps/distance/time	cal. burned

I am pleased with:

What could be improved:

Date: _____

breakfast/lunch/dinner/snacks	carbs	fat	prot.	cal.
Total				

water ☐ ☐ ☐ ☐ ☐ ☐ ☐ ☐

sleep zzz zzz zzz zzz zzz zzz zzz zzz

How do I feel today? ☺ 😐 ☹

activity	sets/reps/distance/time	cal. burned

I am pleased with:	What could be improved:

Date: _____

breakfast/lunch/dinner/snacks	carbs	fat	prot.	cal.
		Total		

water	🥛 🥛 🥛 🥛 🥛 🥛 🥛 🥛	How do I feel today?		
sleep	💤 💤 💤 💤 💤 💤 💤 💤 💤	🙂	😐	☹️

activity	sets/reps/distance/time	cal. burned

I am pleased with:	What could be improved:

Date: _____

breakfast/lunch/dinner/snacks	carbs	fat	prot.	cal.
Total				

water ☐ ☐ ☐ ☐ ☐ ☐ ☐ ☐ ☐
sleep zzz zzz zzz zzz zzz zzz zzz zzz zzz

How do I feel today? ☺ 😐 ☹

activity	sets/reps/distance/time	cal. burned

I am pleased with:	What could be improved:

Date: _____

breakfast/lunch/dinner/snacks	carbs	fat	prot.	cal.
Total				

water	☐ ☐ ☐ ☐ ☐ ☐ ☐ ☐
sleep	zzz zzz zzz zzz zzz zzz zzz zzz zzz

How do I feel today? ☺ 😐 ☹

activity	sets/reps/distance/time	cal. burned

I am pleased with:	What could be improved:

Date: _____

breakfast/lunch/dinner/snacks	carbs	fat	prot.	cal.
Total				

water: ☐ ☐ ☐ ☐ ☐ ☐ ☐ ☐ ☐

sleep: zzz zzz zzz zzz zzz zzz zzz zzz zzz zzz

How do I feel today? 😊 😐 ☹

activity	sets/reps/distance/time	cal. burned

I am pleased with:

What could be improved:

Date: _____

breakfast/lunch/dinner/snacks	carbs	fat	prot.	cal.
Total				

water	🥛 🥛 🥛 🥛 🥛 🥛 🥛 🥛	How do I feel today?
sleep	zzz zzz zzz zzz zzz zzz zzz zzz zzz	😊 😐 ☹

activity	sets/reps/distance/time	cal. burned

I am pleased with:	What could be improved:

Date: _____

breakfast/lunch/dinner/snacks	carbs	fat	prot.	cal.
Total				

water ☐ ☐ ☐ ☐ ☐ ☐ ☐ ☐

sleep zzz zzz zzz zzz zzz zzz zzz zzz zzz

How do I feel today? ☺ 😐 ☹

activity	sets/reps/distance/time	cal. burned

I am pleased with:	What could be improved:

Date: _____

breakfast/lunch/dinner/snacks	carbs	fat	prot.	cal.
Total				

water		How do I feel today?		
sleep		😊	😐	☹

activity	sets/reps/distance/time	cal. burned

I am pleased with:	What could be improved:

Date: _____

breakfast/lunch/dinner/snacks	carbs	fat	prot.	cal.
Total				

water	🥛🥛🥛🥛🥛🥛🥛🥛	How do I feel today?		
sleep	💤💤💤💤💤💤💤💤💤💤	🙂	😐	☹️

activity	sets/reps/distance/time	cal. burned

I am pleased with:	What could be improved:

Date: _____

breakfast/lunch/dinner/snacks	carbs	fat	prot.	cal.
Total				

water		How do I feel today?		
sleep		☺	😐	☹

activity	sets/reps/distance/time	cal. burned

I am pleased with:	What could be improved:

Date: _____

breakfast/lunch/dinner/snacks	carbs	fat	prot.	cal.
Total				

water: ☐ ☐ ☐ ☐ ☐ ☐ ☐ ☐ ☐

sleep: 💤 💤 💤 💤 💤 💤 💤 💤 💤 💤

How do I feel today? 🙂 😐 ☹️

activity	sets/reps/distance/time	cal. burned

I am pleased with:

What could be improved:

Date: _____

breakfast/lunch/dinner/snacks	carbs	fat	prot.	cal.
Total				

water: ☐ ☐ ☐ ☐ ☐ ☐ ☐ ☐
sleep: zzz zzz zzz zzz zzz zzz zzz zzz zzz

How do I feel today? 🙂 😐 ☹

activity	sets/reps/distance/time	cal. burned

I am pleased with:	What could be improved:

Date: _____

breakfast/lunch/dinner/snacks	carbs	fat	prot.	cal.
Total				

water	🥛🥛🥛🥛🥛🥛🥛🥛	How do I feel today?		
sleep	💤💤💤💤💤💤💤💤💤💤	🙂	😐	☹️

activity	sets/reps/distance/time	cal. burned

I am pleased with:	What could be improved:

Date: _____

breakfast/lunch/dinner/snacks	carbs	fat	prot.	cal.
		Total		

water	🥛 🥛 🥛 🥛 🥛 🥛 🥛 🥛	How do I feel today?		
sleep	zzz zzz zzz zzz zzz zzz zzz zzz zzz	🙂	😐	☹️

activity	sets/reps/distance/time	cal. burned

I am pleased with:	What could be improved:

Date: _____

breakfast/lunch/dinner/snacks	carbs	fat	prot.	cal.
Total				

water: ▯ ▯ ▯ ▯ ▯ ▯ ▯ ▯

sleep: zzz zzz zzz zzz zzz zzz zzz zzz zzz

How do I feel today? ☺ 😐 ☹

activity	sets/reps/distance/time	cal. burned

I am pleased with:

What could be improved:

Date: _____

breakfast/lunch/dinner/snacks	carbs	fat	prot.	cal.
Total				

water	🥛 🥛 🥛 🥛 🥛 🥛 🥛 🥛	How do I feel today?		
sleep	zzz zzz zzz zzz zzz zzz zzz zzz zzz	🙂	😐	☹️

activity	sets/reps/distance/time	cal. burned

I am pleased with:	What could be improved:

Date: _____

breakfast/lunch/dinner/snacks	carbs	fat	prot.	cal.
Total				

water ☐☐☐☐☐☐☐☐☐

sleep zzz zzz zzz zzz zzz zzz zzz zzz zzz

How do I feel today? 😊 | 😐 | ☹️

activity	sets/reps/distance/time	cal. burned

I am pleased with:

What could be improved:

Date: _____

breakfast/lunch/dinner/snacks	carbs	fat	prot.	cal.
Total				

water	🥛 🥛 🥛 🥛 🥛 🥛 🥛 🥛	How do I feel today?		
sleep	zzz zzz zzz zzz zzz zzz zzz zzz zzz	🙂	😐	☹️

activity	sets/reps/distance/time	cal. burned

I am pleased with:	What could be improved:

Date: _____

breakfast/lunch/dinner/snacks	carbs	fat	prot.	cal.
Total				

water 🥛🥛🥛🥛🥛🥛🥛🥛

sleep 💤💤💤💤💤💤💤💤💤

How do I feel today? 🙂 😐 ☹️

activity	sets/reps/distance/time	cal. burned

I am pleased with:

What could be improved:

Date: _____

breakfast/lunch/dinner/snacks	carbs	fat	prot.	cal.
Total				

water	🥛 🥛 🥛 🥛 🥛 🥛 🥛 🥛	How do I feel today?		
sleep	💤 💤 💤 💤 💤 💤 💤 💤 💤	🙂	😐	☹️

activity	sets/reps/distance/time	cal. burned

I am pleased with:	What could be improved:

Date: _____

breakfast/lunch/dinner/snacks	carbs	fat	prot.	cal.
Total				

water	🥛 🥛 🥛 🥛 🥛 🥛 🥛 🥛	How do I feel today?		
sleep	💤 💤 💤 💤 💤 💤 💤 💤 💤 💤	🙂	😐	☹️

activity	sets/reps/distance/time	cal. burned

I am pleased with:	What could be improved:

Date: _____

breakfast/lunch/dinner/snacks	carbs	fat	prot.	cal.
Total				

water	🥛 🥛 🥛 🥛 🥛 🥛 🥛 🥛	How do I feel today?		
sleep	💤 💤 💤 💤 💤 💤 💤 💤 💤	🙂	😐	☹️

activity	sets/reps/distance/time	cal. burned

I am pleased with:	What could be improved:

Date: _____

breakfast/lunch/dinner/snacks	carbs	fat	prot.	cal.
Total				

water ☐ ☐ ☐ ☐ ☐ ☐ ☐ ☐ ☐ ☐

sleep 💤 💤 💤 💤 💤 💤 💤 💤 💤 💤

How do I feel today? 😊 😐 ☹

activity	sets/reps/distance/time	cal. burned

I am pleased with:

What could be improved:

Date: _____

breakfast/lunch/dinner/snacks	carbs	fat	prot.	cal.
Total				

water	🥛🥛🥛🥛🥛🥛🥛🥛	How do I feel today?		
sleep	💤💤💤💤💤💤💤💤	🙂	😐	☹️

activity	sets/reps/distance/time	cal. burned

I am pleased with:	What could be improved:

Date: _____

breakfast/lunch/dinner/snacks	carbs	fat	prot.	cal.
	Total			

water 🥛🥛🥛🥛🥛🥛🥛🥛

sleep 💤💤💤💤💤💤💤💤💤💤

How do I feel today? 🙂 😐 ☹

activity	sets/reps/distance/time	cal. burned

I am pleased with:	What could be improved:

Date: _____

breakfast/lunch/dinner/snacks	carbs	fat	prot.	cal.
	Total			

water	🥛 🥛 🥛 🥛 🥛 🥛 🥛 🥛
sleep	zzz zzz zzz zzz zzz zzz zzz zzz zzz

How do I feel today? 🙂 😐 ☹️

activity	sets/reps/distance/time	cal. burned

I am pleased with:	What could be improved:

Date: _____

breakfast/lunch/dinner/snacks	carbs	fat	prot.	cal.
Total				

water ☐ ☐ ☐ ☐ ☐ ☐ ☐ ☐ ☐
sleep zzz zzz zzz zzz zzz zzz zzz zzz zzz zzz

How do I feel today? ☺ 😐 ☹

activity	sets/reps/distance/time	cal. burned

I am pleased with:	What could be improved:

Date: _____

breakfast/lunch/dinner/snacks	carbs	fat	prot.	cal.
Total				

water	🥛🥛🥛🥛🥛🥛🥛🥛	How do I feel today?		
sleep	zzz zzz zzz zzz zzz zzz zzz zzz zzz	🙂	😐	☹️

activity	sets/reps/distance/time	cal. burned

I am pleased with:	What could be improved:

Date: _____

breakfast/lunch/dinner/snacks	carbs	fat	prot.	cal.
Total				

water ▢▢▢▢▢▢▢▢▢

sleep 💤💤💤💤💤💤💤💤💤💤

How do I feel today? 😊 😐 ☹️

activity	sets/reps/distance/time	cal. burned

I am pleased with:	What could be improved:

Date: _____

breakfast/lunch/dinner/snacks	carbs	fat	prot.	cal.
Total				

water ☐☐☐☐☐☐☐☐

sleep zzz zzz zzz zzz zzz zzz zzz zzz zzz

How do I feel today? 😊 😐 ☹

activity	sets/reps/distance/time	cal. burned

I am pleased with:

What could be improved:

Date: _____

breakfast/lunch/dinner/snacks	carbs	fat	prot.	cal.
	Total			

water: ☐ ☐ ☐ ☐ ☐ ☐ ☐ ☐

sleep: zzz zzz zzz zzz zzz zzz zzz zzz zzz

How do I feel today? 😊 😐 ☹

activity	sets/reps/distance/time	cal. burned

I am pleased with:	What could be improved:

Date:_____

breakfast/lunch/dinner/snacks	carbs	fat	prot.	cal.
Total				

water	🥛 🥛 🥛 🥛 🥛 🥛 🥛 🥛	How do I feel today?		
sleep	zzz zzz zzz zzz zzz zzz zzz zzz zzz	😊	😐	☹️

activity	sets/reps/distance/time	cal. burned

I am pleased with:	What could be improved:

Date: _____

breakfast/lunch/dinner/snacks	carbs	fat	prot.	cal.
	Total			

water ▯ ▯ ▯ ▯ ▯ ▯ ▯ ▯

sleep zzz zzz zzz zzz zzz zzz zzz zzz zzz

How do I feel today? ☺ 😐 ☹

activity	sets/reps/distance/time	cal. burned

I am pleased with:	What could be improved:

Date: _____

breakfast/lunch/dinner/snacks	carbs	fat	prot.	cal.
Total				

water	☐ ☐ ☐ ☐ ☐ ☐ ☐ ☐	How do I feel today?	
sleep	zzz zzz zzz zzz zzz zzz zzz zzz zzz	☺ ☺ ☹	

activity	sets/reps/distance/time	cal. burned

I am pleased with:	What could be improved:

Date: _____

breakfast/lunch/dinner/snacks	carbs	fat	prot.	cal.
Total				

water ☐ ☐ ☐ ☐ ☐ ☐ ☐ ☐ ☐ ☐

sleep 💤 💤 💤 💤 💤 💤 💤 💤 💤 💤

How do I feel today? 🙂 😐 🙁

activity	sets/reps/distance/time	cal. burned

I am pleased with:	What could be improved:

Date: _____

breakfast/lunch/dinner/snacks	carbs	fat	prot.	cal.
Total				

water	☐ ☐ ☐ ☐ ☐ ☐ ☐ ☐	How do I feel today?	
sleep	zzz zzz zzz zzz zzz zzz zzz zzz zzz	😊 😐 ☹	

activity	sets/reps/distance/time	cal. burned

I am pleased with:	What could be improved:

Date: _____

breakfast/lunch/dinner/snacks	carbs	fat	prot.	cal.
Total				

water	🥛 🥛 🥛 🥛 🥛 🥛 🥛 🥛	How do I feel today?		
sleep	zzz zzz zzz zzz zzz zzz zzz zzz zzz	🙂	😐	☹️

activity	sets/reps/distance/time	cal. burned

I am pleased with:	What could be improved:

Date: _____

breakfast/lunch/dinner/snacks	carbs	fat	prot.	cal.
Total				

water	🥛 🥛 🥛 🥛 🥛 🥛 🥛 🥛	How do I feel today?		
sleep	💤 💤 💤 💤 💤 💤 💤 💤 💤	🙂	😐	☹️

activity	sets/reps/distance/time	cal. burned

I am pleased with:	What could be improved:

Date: _____

breakfast/lunch/dinner/snacks	carbs	fat	prot.	cal.
	Total			

water: ☐ ☐ ☐ ☐ ☐ ☐ ☐ ☐
sleep: zzz zzz zzz zzz zzz zzz zzz zzz zzz zzz

How do I feel today? ☺ 😐 ☹

activity	sets/reps/distance/time	cal. burned

I am pleased with:	What could be improved:

Date: _____

breakfast/lunch/dinner/snacks	carbs	fat	prot.	cal.
Total				

water	☐ ☐ ☐ ☐ ☐ ☐ ☐ ☐	How do I feel today?		
sleep	zzz zzz zzz zzz zzz zzz zzz zzz	☺	😐	☹

activity	sets/reps/distance/time	cal. burned

I am pleased with:	What could be improved:

Date: _____

breakfast/lunch/dinner/snacks	carbs	fat	prot.	cal.
Total				

water: ☐ ☐ ☐ ☐ ☐ ☐ ☐ ☐

sleep: zzz zzz zzz zzz zzz zzz zzz zzz zzz zzz

How do I feel today? 🙂 😐 ☹

activity	sets/reps/distance/time	cal. burned

I am pleased with:	What could be improved:

Date: _____

breakfast/lunch/dinner/snacks	carbs	fat	prot.	cal.
Total				

water	☐ ☐ ☐ ☐ ☐ ☐ ☐ ☐	How do I feel today?		
sleep	zzz zzz zzz zzz zzz zzz zzz zzz zzz	☺	😐	☹

activity	sets/reps/distance/time	cal. burned

I am pleased with:	What could be improved:

Date: _____

breakfast/lunch/dinner/snacks	carbs	fat	prot.	cal.
Total				

water ☐ ☐ ☐ ☐ ☐ ☐ ☐ ☐

sleep zzz zzz zzz zzz zzz zzz zzz zzz zzz zzz

How do I feel today? 😊 😐 ☹

activity	sets/reps/distance/time	cal. burned

I am pleased with:	What could be improved:

Date: _____

breakfast/lunch/dinner/snacks	carbs	fat	prot.	cal.
Total				

water	🥛 🥛 🥛 🥛 🥛 🥛 🥛 🥛
sleep	💤 💤 💤 💤 💤 💤 💤 💤 💤

How do I feel today? 😊 | 😐 | ☹️

activity	sets/reps/distance/time	cal. burned

I am pleased with:	What could be improved:

Date: _____

breakfast/lunch/dinner/snacks	carbs	fat	prot.	cal.
	Total			

water		How do I feel today?		
sleep		☺	😐	☹

activity	sets/reps/distance/time	cal. burned

I am pleased with:	What could be improved:

Date: _____

breakfast/lunch/dinner/snacks	carbs	fat	prot.	cal.
Total				

water	🥛 🥛 🥛 🥛 🥛 🥛 🥛 🥛	How do I feel today?
sleep	💤 💤 💤 💤 💤 💤 💤 💤 💤	🙂 😐 ☹️

activity	sets/reps/distance/time	cal. burned

I am pleased with:	What could be improved:

Date: _____

breakfast/lunch/dinner/snacks	carbs	fat	prot.	cal.
Total				

water ▢▢▢▢▢▢▢▢▢

sleep 💤💤💤💤💤💤💤💤💤💤

How do I feel today? 🙂 😐 🙁

activity	sets/reps/distance/time	cal. burned

I am pleased with:	What could be improved:

Date: _____

breakfast/lunch/dinner/snacks	carbs	fat	prot.	cal.
Total				

			How do I feel today?		
water	🥛🥛🥛🥛🥛🥛🥛🥛		☺	😐	☹
sleep	💤💤💤💤💤💤💤💤💤💤				

activity	sets/reps/distance/time	cal. burned

I am pleased with:	What could be improved:

Date: _____

breakfast/lunch/dinner/snacks	carbs	fat	prot.	cal.
	Total			

water	▯ ▯ ▯ ▯ ▯ ▯ ▯ ▯	How do I feel today?		
sleep	zzz zzz zzz zzz zzz zzz zzz zzz zzz zzz	🙂	😐	☹

activity	sets/reps/distance/time	cal. burned

I am pleased with:	What could be improved:

Date: _____

breakfast/lunch/dinner/snacks	carbs	fat	prot.	cal.
Total				

water	🥛 🥛 🥛 🥛 🥛 🥛 🥛 🥛	How do I feel today?		
sleep	zzz zzz zzz zzz zzz zzz zzz zzz zzz	🙂	😐	🙁

activity	sets/reps/distance/time	cal. burned

I am pleased with:	What could be improved:

Date: _____

breakfast/lunch/dinner/snacks	carbs	fat	prot.	cal.
Total				

water	🥛🥛🥛🥛🥛🥛🥛🥛🥛🥛	How do I feel today?		
sleep	💤💤💤💤💤💤💤💤💤💤	🙂	😐	☹️

activity	sets/reps/distance/time	cal. burned

I am pleased with:	What could be improved:

Date: _____

breakfast/lunch/dinner/snacks	carbs	fat	prot.	cal.
Total				

water	🥛 🥛 🥛 🥛 🥛 🥛 🥛 🥛	How do I feel today?		
sleep	💤 💤 💤 💤 💤 💤 💤 💤 💤	🙂	😐	☹️

activity	sets/reps/distance/time	cal. burned

I am pleased with:	What could be improved:

Date: _____

breakfast/lunch/dinner/snacks	carbs	fat	prot.	cal.
Total				

water ☐ ☐ ☐ ☐ ☐ ☐ ☐ ☐ ☐

sleep 💤 💤 💤 💤 💤 💤 💤 💤 💤 💤

How do I feel today? 🙂 😐 ☹️

activity	sets/reps/distance/time	cal. burned

I am pleased with:	What could be improved:

Date: _____

breakfast/lunch/dinner/snacks	carbs	fat	prot.	cal.
Total				

water	🥛🥛🥛🥛🥛🥛🥛🥛	How do I feel today?		
sleep	zzz zzz zzz zzz zzz zzz zzz zzz zzz	☺	😐	☹

activity	sets/reps/distance/time	cal. burned

I am pleased with:	What could be improved:

Date: _____

breakfast/lunch/dinner/snacks	carbs	fat	prot.	cal.
Total				

water ▯▯▯▯▯▯▯▯▯
sleep zzz zzz zzz zzz zzz zzz zzz zzz zzz zzz

How do I feel today? ☺ 😐 ☹

activity	sets/reps/distance/time	cal. burned

I am pleased with:

What could be improved:

Date: _____

breakfast/lunch/dinner/snacks	carbs	fat	prot.	cal.
	Total			

water 🥛🥛🥛🥛🥛🥛🥛🥛

sleep 💤💤💤💤💤💤💤💤💤

How do I feel today? 😊 😐 ☹️

activity	sets/reps/distance/time	cal. burned

I am pleased with:

What could be improved:

Date: _____

breakfast/lunch/dinner/snacks	carbs	fat	prot.	cal.
	Total			

water: ☐ ☐ ☐ ☐ ☐ ☐ ☐ ☐

sleep: zzz zzz zzz zzz zzz zzz zzz zzz zzz zzz

How do I feel today? 😊 😐 ☹

activity	sets/reps/distance/time	cal. burned

I am pleased with:	What could be improved:

Date: _____

breakfast/lunch/dinner/snacks	carbs	fat	prot.	cal.
Total				

water ☐☐☐☐☐☐☐☐

sleep 💤💤💤💤💤💤💤💤💤

How do I feel today? 😊 😐 ☹

activity	sets/reps/distance/time	cal. burned

I am pleased with:

What could be improved:

Date: _____

breakfast/lunch/dinner/snacks	carbs	fat	prot.	cal.
Total				

water ▭▭▭▭▭▭▭▭▭▭

sleep zzz zzz zzz zzz zzz zzz zzz zzz zzz zzz

How do I feel today? ☺ 😐 ☹

activity	sets/reps/distance/time	cal. burned

I am pleased with:	What could be improved:

Date: _____

breakfast/lunch/dinner/snacks	carbs	fat	prot.	cal.
Total				

water	🥛 🥛 🥛 🥛 🥛 🥛 🥛 🥛	How do I feel today?		
sleep	zzz zzz zzz zzz zzz zzz zzz zzz zzz	🙂	😐	☹

activity	sets/reps/distance/time	cal. burned

I am pleased with:	What could be improved:

Date: _____

breakfast/lunch/dinner/snacks	carbs	fat	prot.	cal.
Total				

water	🥛 🥛 🥛 🥛 🥛 🥛 🥛 🥛	How do I feel today?		
sleep	zzz zzz zzz zzz zzz zzz zzz zzz zzz	😊	😐	☹

activity	sets/reps/distance/time	cal. burned

I am pleased with:	What could be improved:

Date: _____

breakfast/lunch/dinner/snacks	carbs	fat	prot.	cal.
Total				

water	🥤 🥤 🥤 🥤 🥤 🥤 🥤 🥤
sleep	zzz zzz zzz zzz zzz zzz zzz zzz zzz

How do I feel today? 😊 😐 ☹

activity	sets/reps/distance/time	cal. burned

I am pleased with:	What could be improved:

Date: _____

breakfast/lunch/dinner/snacks	carbs	fat	prot.	cal.
Total				

water	🥛 🥛 🥛 🥛 🥛 🥛 🥛 🥛	How do I feel today?		
sleep	zzz zzz zzz zzz zzz zzz zzz zzz zzz zzz	😊	😐	☹️

activity	sets/reps/distance/time	cal. burned

I am pleased with:	What could be improved:

Date: _____

breakfast/lunch/dinner/snacks	carbs	fat	prot.	cal.
	Total			

water 🥛🥛🥛🥛🥛🥛🥛🥛
sleep 💤💤💤💤💤💤💤💤💤💤

How do I feel today? 😊 | 😐 | ☹️

activity	sets/reps/distance/time	cal. burned

I am pleased with:	What could be improved:

Date: _____

breakfast/lunch/dinner/snacks	carbs	fat	prot.	cal.
	Total			

water: ☐ ☐ ☐ ☐ ☐ ☐ ☐ ☐

sleep: 💤 💤 💤 💤 💤 💤 💤 💤 💤

How do I feel today? 😊 😐 ☹

activity	sets/reps/distance/time	cal. burned

I am pleased with:

What could be improved:

Date: _____

breakfast/lunch/dinner/snacks	carbs	fat	prot.	cal.
Total				

water	🥛🥛🥛🥛🥛🥛🥛🥛	How do I feel today?		
sleep	zzz zzz zzz zzz zzz zzz zzz zzz zzz	😊	😐	☹️

activity	sets/reps/distance/time	cal. burned

I am pleased with:	What could be improved:

Date: _____

breakfast/lunch/dinner/snacks	carbs	fat	prot.	cal.
Total				

water	🥛 🥛 🥛 🥛 🥛 🥛 🥛 🥛	How do I feel today?		
sleep	💤 💤 💤 💤 💤 💤 💤 💤 💤 💤	🙂	😐	☹️

activity	sets/reps/distance/time	cal. burned

I am pleased with:	What could be improved:

Date: _____

breakfast/lunch/dinner/snacks	carbs	fat	prot.	cal.
	Total			

water	🥛 🥛 🥛 🥛 🥛 🥛 🥛 🥛
sleep	💤 💤 💤 💤 💤 💤 💤 💤 💤

How do I feel today? 😊 😐 ☹️

activity	sets/reps/distance/time	cal. burned

I am pleased with:	What could be improved:

Date: _____

breakfast/lunch/dinner/snacks	carbs	fat	prot.	cal.
Total				

water ▯ ▯ ▯ ▯ ▯ ▯ ▯ ▯ ▯ ▯

sleep zzz zzz zzz zzz zzz zzz zzz zzz zzz zzz

How do I feel today? ☺ 😐 ☹

activity	sets/reps/distance/time	cal. burned

I am pleased with:	What could be improved:

Date: _____

breakfast/lunch/dinner/snacks	carbs	fat	prot.	cal.
	Total			

		How do I feel today?
water	☐ ☐ ☐ ☐ ☐ ☐ ☐ ☐	😊 😐 ☹
sleep	zzz zzz zzz zzz zzz zzz zzz zzz zzz	

activity	sets/reps/distance/time	cal. burned

I am pleased with:	What could be improved:

Date: _____

breakfast/lunch/dinner/snacks	carbs	fat	prot.	cal.
Total				

water ☐☐☐☐☐☐☐☐☐☐

sleep zzz zzz zzz zzz zzz zzz zzz zzz zzz zzz

How do I feel today? ☺ 😐 ☹

activity	sets/reps/distance/time	cal. burned

I am pleased with:	What could be improved:

Date: _____

breakfast/lunch/dinner/snacks	carbs	fat	prot.	cal.
Total				

water	🥛 🥛 🥛 🥛 🥛 🥛 🥛 🥛
sleep	💤 💤 💤 💤 💤 💤 💤 💤 💤

How do I feel today? ☺ 😐 ☹

activity	sets/reps/distance/time	cal. burned

I am pleased with:	What could be improved:

Date: _____

breakfast/lunch/dinner/snacks	carbs	fat	prot.	cal.
	Total			

water	🥛 🥛 🥛 🥛 🥛 🥛 🥛 🥛	How do I feel today?		
sleep	zzz zzz zzz zzz zzz zzz zzz zzz zzz zzz	😊	😐	☹️

activity	sets/reps/distance/time	cal. burned

I am pleased with:	What could be improved:

Date: _____

breakfast/lunch/dinner/snacks	carbs	fat	prot.	cal.
	Total			

water	🥛 🥛 🥛 🥛 🥛 🥛 🥛 🥛	How do I feel today?		
sleep	zzz zzz zzz zzz zzz zzz zzz zzz zzz	😊	😐	☹️

activity	sets/reps/distance/time	cal. burned

I am pleased with:	What could be improved:

Date: _____

breakfast/lunch/dinner/snacks	carbs	fat	prot.	cal.
Total				

		How do I feel today?		
water	🥛🥛🥛🥛🥛🥛🥛🥛🥛🥛	☺	😐	☹
sleep	💤💤💤💤💤💤💤💤💤💤			

activity	sets/reps/distance/time	cal. burned

I am pleased with:	What could be improved:

Date: _____

breakfast/lunch/dinner/snacks	carbs	fat	prot.	cal.
	Total			

water

sleep

How do I feel today? 😊 😐 ☹

activity	sets/reps/distance/time	cal. burned

I am pleased with:

What could be improved:

Date: _____

breakfast/lunch/dinner/snacks	carbs	fat	prot.	cal.
Total				

water ☐☐☐☐☐☐☐☐ How do I feel today? ☺ 😐 ☹

sleep zzz zzz zzz zzz zzz zzz zzz zzz zzz

activity	sets/reps/distance/time	cal. burned

I am pleased with:	What could be improved:

Date: _____

breakfast/lunch/dinner/snacks	carbs	fat	prot.	cal.
Total				

water	🥛 🥛 🥛 🥛 🥛 🥛 🥛 🥛	How do I feel today?		
sleep	zzz zzz zzz zzz zzz zzz zzz zzz zzz	🙂	😐	☹

activity	sets/reps/distance/time	cal. burned

I am pleased with:	What could be improved:

Date: _____

breakfast/lunch/dinner/snacks	carbs	fat	prot.	cal.
Total				

water	🥛 🥛 🥛 🥛 🥛 🥛 🥛 🥛	How do I feel today?
sleep	zzz zzz zzz zzz zzz zzz zzz zzz zzz zzz	🙂 😐 ☹

activity	sets/reps/distance/time	cal. burned

I am pleased with:	What could be improved:

www.ingramcontent.com/pod-product-compliance
Lightning Source LLC
Chambersburg PA
CBHW070425220526
45466CB00004B/1545